20 Questions & Answers
About Metastatic Castration-Resistant Prostate Cancer

Pamela Ellsworth, MD

Professor of Urology
UMass Memorial Medical Center
University of Massachusetts Medical
Worcester, MA

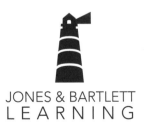

JONES & BARTLETT
LEARNING

World Headquarters
Jones & Bartlett Learning
5 Wall Street
Burlington, MA 01803
978-443-5000
info@jblearning.com
www.jblearning.com

Jones & Bartlett Learning books and products are available through most bookstores and online booksellers. To contact Jones & Bartlett Learning directly, call 800-832-0034, fax 978-443-8000, or visit our website, www.jblearning.com.

Substantial discounts on bulk quantities of Jones & Bartlett Learning publications are available to corporations, professional associations, and other qualified organizations. For details and specific discount information, contact the special sales department at Jones & Bartlett Learning via the above contact information or send an email to specialsales@jblearning.com.

Production Credits

Executive Acquisitions Editor: Nancy Anastasi Duffy
Production Assistant: Alex Schab
Manufacturing and Inventory Control Supervisor: Amy Bacus
Composition: Jason Miranda, Spoke & Wheel
Cover Design: Kristin E. Parker

Photo Research and Permissions Coordinator: Lauren Miller
Cover Image: Top: © PhotoDisc, Bottom Right: © PhotoDisc, Bottom Left: © Doug Menuez/PhotoDisc
Printing and Binding: Edwards Brothers Malloy
Cover Printing: Edwards Brothers Malloy

ISBN: 978-1-284-04836-0

6048

Printed in the United States of America
18 17 16 15 14   10 9 8 7 6 5 4 3 2 1

CONTENTS

Prostate cancer is the most commonly diagnosed solid organ cancer in the United States and is the second leading cause of death among men in the United States. In 2012, there were approximately 240,000 new diagnoses of prostate cancer and an estimated 28,000 deaths resulted from the cancer. Prostate cancer deaths are typically the result of metastatic castration-resistant prostate cancer (mCRPC). Historically, men tended to die within 2 years of developing mCRPC. However, the recent development of several new therapies has provided hope of improved survival rates for men with mCRPC. As of yet, however, these therapies have not been able to cure the cancer and so more research is needed.

ACKNOWLEDGMENTS

A special thank you to Timothy Haaga, MD, who provided the radiologic images and information on the use of the various radiologic studies. He is a resident physician in the Diagnostic Imaging Department of Rhode Island Hospital and Brown University Warren Alpert School of Medicine. He is pursuing a career in Diagnostic Neuroradiology and will complete his Neuroradiology Fellowship at the Weill Cornell Medical College of Cornell University.

PART ONE

The Basics

What is metastatic castration-resistant
prostate cancer (mCRPC)?

What are the signs and symptoms of mCRPC?

I thought "castration" meant removal of the testicles,
but I still have mine. I am on castration medications;
can I be castrated by them?

More...

Cancer

Abnormal and uncontrolled growth of cells in the body that can spread, injure areas of the body, and cause death.

Testosterone

The male hormone or androgen that is produced primarily by the testes and is needed for sexual function and fertility.

Bilateral orchiectomy

Surgical removal of both testicles.

Androgen deprivation therapy (ADT)

Therapy designed to lower the testosterone level in the body by preventing its production (most commonly, LHRH agonists/antagonists).

LHRH agonist

A class of drugs that works at the level of the brain, which initially overstimulates the brain before suppressing the production of testosterone by the testicles. This short period of overstimulation can increase the testosterone level and cause bone pain in patients with bone metastases, known as the "flare phenomenon."

1. What is metastatic castration-resistant prostate cancer (mCRPC)?

Castration-resistant prostate cancer (CRPC) is a term that applies to prostate **cancer** that has progressed despite the use of therapies to lower the **testosterone** level in the body. These therapies include **bilateral orchiectomy** (surgical removal of the testicles) and **androgen deprivation therapy** (stopping the testicles from producing testosterone, **LHRH agonist** and **LHRH antagonist**; it is abbreviated as ADT). **Anti-androgens** are hormonal therapies designed to block testosterone from stimulating prostate cancer cells to grow. However, in men with CRPC, the prostate cancer still responds to even the low levels of testosterone present on anti-androgen therapy.

In clinical terms, CRPC is the progression of prostate cancer in patients with castrate levels of testosterone (< 20 to 50 ng/mL). To put this in perspective, mid-normal range testosterone levels in young, healthy men are 400–700 ng/mL, while normal testosterone levels are slightly lower in older men. This progression initially may be an increase in prostate-specific **antigen** (PSA) levels (**PSA progression**) or may be associated with metastases (the spread of prostate cancer to areas in the body outside of the prostate **gland**, commonly the **lymph nodes**, which are involved in the production of **lymph,** and bones). This is referred to as metastatic castration-resistant prostate cancer (mCRPC). See **Figure 1** through **Figure 4**.

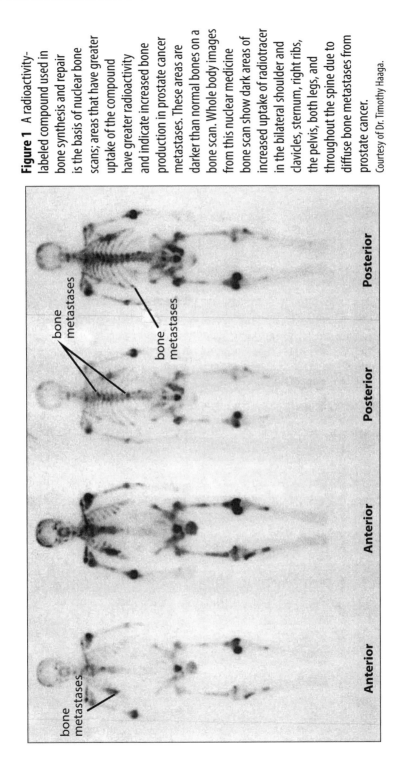

Figure 1 A radioactivity-labeled compound used in bone synthesis and repair is the basis of nuclear bone scans; areas that have greater uptake of the compound have greater radioactivity and indicate increased bone production in prostate cancer metastases. These areas are darker than normal bones on a bone scan. Whole body images from this nuclear medicine bone scan show dark areas of increased uptake of radiotracer in the bilateral shoulder and clavicles, sternum, right ribs, the pelvis, both legs, and throughout the spine due to diffuse bone metastases from prostate cancer.
Courtesy of Dr. Timothy Haaga.

LHRH antagonist

A form of hormone therapy that works at the level of the brain to directly suppress the production of testosterone without initially raising the testosterone level. There is no flare reaction.

Anti-androgen

A medication that eliminates or reduces the presence or activity of androgens.

Antigen

A substance that stimulates the body to produce an antibody.

PSA progression

Rising PSA levels despite therapy to treat prostate cancer.

Gland

A structure or organ that produces substances that affect other areas of the body.

Lymph node(s)

Small, bean-shaped glands that are found throughout the body. Lymph fluid passes through the lymph nodes, which filter out bacteria, cancer cells, and toxic chemicals.

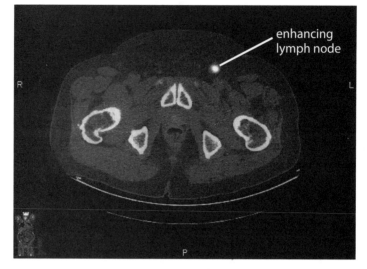

Figure 2 The increased use of glucose by cancerous cells compared to normal tissue is the basis of PET imaging where concentrated radioactive glucose accumulates preferentially in primary tumors and metastases. PET images are fused with CT images to see what anatomical structure corresponds to the increased uptake. Fused axial PET-CT image shows a very hypermetabolic ("hot") lymph node to the left groin due to presumed prostate cancer metastasis to a lymph node.
Courtesy of Dr. Timothy Haaga.

The Prostate Cancer Clinical Trials Working Group defines asymptomatic nonmetastatic castration-resistant prostate cancer as an increase in PSA level both 2 ng/mL above and 25% higher than **PSA nadir** (the lowest level of PSA a patient exhibited during treatment). This must then be confirmed by a second PSA level test at least 3 weeks later. In addition, there must be no radiographic evidence of metastatic disease.

In order to meet the European Association of Urology's (EAU) definition of CRPC, the following must occur:

- The patient must possess a testosterone level of less than 50 ng/mL.

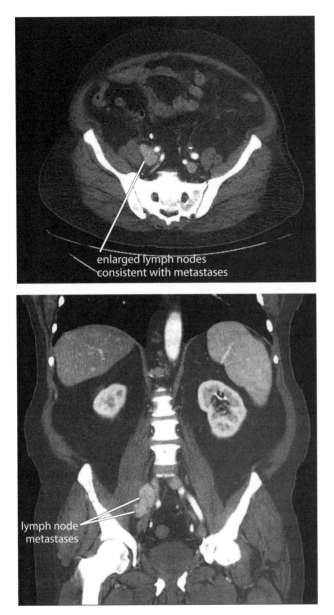

Lymph

A clear fluid that is found throughout the body. Lymph fluid helps fight infections.

PSA nadir

The lowest value that the PSA level reaches during a particular treatment.

THE BASICS

Figures 3 and 4 Normal lymph nodes do not grow or have significant blood flow to them unless affected by infection or tumor. The use of IV contrast on CT scan helps to detect blood flow in tissue by showing tissue enhancement or "lighting up" with contrast. These images from an IV contrast–enhanced CT scan show enhancing, enlarged right common iliac nodes that had enlarged compared to a prior CT scan and were highly suspicious for metastases to pelvic lymph nodes from prostate cancer.
Courtesy of Dr. Timothy Haaga.

- Tests must confirm three consecutive increases in PSA levels, 1 week apart, resulting in two 50% increases over the nadir.
- The patient has to have been receiving combination hormonal therapy (androgen agonist/antagonist + anti-androgen) and have stopped receiving the anti-androgen for 4 to 6 weeks (depending on the anti-androgen used), with an increasing PSA thereafter.
- There must be evidence of the progression of bone metastases or the development of two or more new lesions, bone metastases, or lymph node metastases at least 2 cm in diameter.

Men with CRPC might only show increasing PSA levels or evidence that the cancer has metastasized, typically, to the pelvic lymph nodes and bones.

Metastatic castration-resistant prostate cancer (mCRPC)

Prostate cancer that continues to progress despite ADT and its resultant low (< 20–50 ng/dL) testosterone level and has spread to an area outside of the prostate gland, such as the bones or lymph nodes.

Metastatic cancer

Cancer that has spread to another area in the body from the organ or structure in which it first arose.

Men with CRPC might only show increasing PSA levels or evidence that the cancer has metastasized, typically, to the pelvic lymph nodes and bones, which is known as **metastatic castration-resistant prostate cancer (mCRPC)**. If the patient is receiving androgen deprivation therapy, the PSA level and PSA doubling time (the estimated amount of time it takes for the PSA level to double) can predict that scans will show **metastatic cancer** in the bone. Studies have demonstrated that a PSA level higher than 10 ng/mL while on ADT is associated with the cancer spreading more rapidly to the bone.

2. What are the signs and symptoms of mCRPC?

Not all men with mCRPC initially have **signs** or **symptoms**. In some men, the initial presentation of mCRPC is a rising PSA level while they are receiving androgen deprivation therapy with asymptomatic metastatic disease. Symptoms of mCRPC reflect the spread of prostate cancer to various parts of the body.

Growth of the prostate cancer within the prostate may lead to cancerous enlargement of the prostate, causing the patient to have trouble urinating (a weak stream, straining to urinate, feeling of incomplete emptying, blood in the urine, and inability to urinate). If the prostate cancer spreads into the bladder, it could lead to obstruction of the **ureters** (the tubes that drain the urine from the kidneys to the bladder), causing back pain, nausea, vomiting, and abnormal kidney function.

When prostate cancer spreads to the bones, pain is the most common symptom (see Figure 1). However, when prostate cancer spreads to the bone, it also weakens the bone, making it more susceptible to fracture. The most commonly affected bones include the spine, ribs, hip, and **femur**; however, other bones can also be affected. If the cancer spreads to the spine, it can cause **spinal cord compression**, which may cause weakness, the inability to walk, and urinary and fecal incontinence (loss of control of urine and stool).

Prostate cancer can also spread to the lymph nodes (**Figures 2 and 3**). If the lymph nodes are extensively affected, the patient may experience swelling of the legs and the obstruction of the ureters.

General symptoms in advanced prostate cancer can include loss of energy (fatigue), weight loss, and loss of appetite.

Sign

Objective evidence of a disease; something that the doctor identifies.

Symptom

Subjective evidence of a disease; something a patient describes, such as pain in the bones.

Ureters

The tubes that drain the urine from the kidneys to the bladder.

Femur

The thigh bone.

Spinal cord compression

Compression of the spinal cord by bone, tumor, or other causes with symptoms ranging from temporary numbness to permanent paralysis of the body below the level of the compression.

General symptoms in advanced prostate cancer can include loss of energy (fatigue), weight loss, and loss of appetite.

3. I thought "castration" meant removal of the testicles, but I still have mine. I am on castration medications; can I be castrated by them?

Castration

The removal of both testicles (bilateral orchiectomy).

Organ

Tissues in the body (e.g., kidneys, bladder, heart) that work together to perform a specific function.

Adrenal glands

Glands located above each kidney. These glands produce several different hormones, including sex hormones.

Orchiectomy

The surgical procedure that removes the testicle(s).

Hormones

Substances (estrogens and androgens) responsible for secondary sex characteristics (hair growth and voice change in men) and function of sexual organs.

Hypothalamus

The region of brain that produces LHRH.

Pituitary gland

The region of the brain that produces LH.

The definition of **castration** is "removal of the testicles from a male." The result of removing the testicles is a marked decrease in the testosterone level in the body. However, the testosterone level does not go to "0" after the testicles are removed, as other **organs** in the body, the **adrenal glands** (small organs located just above the kidneys on both sides of the body), produce small amounts of testosterone. Despite this, the majority of testosterone is produced by the testicles, and removing them will cause the body's testosterone level to drop below 20 to 50 ng/mL. However, ADT can result in testosterone levels that match those resulting from castration. When this occurs, it is known as "medical castration." With regular administration of therapy, medical castration is as effective as an **orchiectomy**.

The medications that are used to lower the testosterone level affect the **hormone** that stimulates the testicles to produce testosterone, which is known as luteinizing hormone (LH). LH levels in the body are high when testosterone levels are low and low when testosterone levels are high. However, in order to produce LH when testosterone levels are low, the **hypothalamus** first produces luteinizing hormone-releasing hormone (LHRH) to stimulate the **pituitary gland**. LHRH stimulates the pituitary gland to produce LH. LH stimulates the testicles to produce testosterone. The amount of testosterone produced negatively affects production of LHRH; the more testosterone that is produced, the lower the LHRH level. This cycle of stimuli is known as a feedback loop, in which organ A stimulates organ B to produce a chemical which in turn affects organ A's stimulation of organ B. See **Figure 5**.

In order to impact the production of LH, one of two different LHRH-directed therapies are used: **LHRH agonists** or LHRH antagonists. When an LHRH agonist is administered, there is an initial increase in the production of LH and a subsequent rise of testosterone levels. This super stimulation in turn tells the brain to

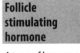

LHRH agonist

A class of drugs that works at the level of the brain, which initially overstimulates the brain before suppressing the production of testosterone by the testicles. This short period of overstimulation can increase the testosterone level and cause bone pain in patients with bone metastases, known as the "flare phenomenon."

THE BASICS

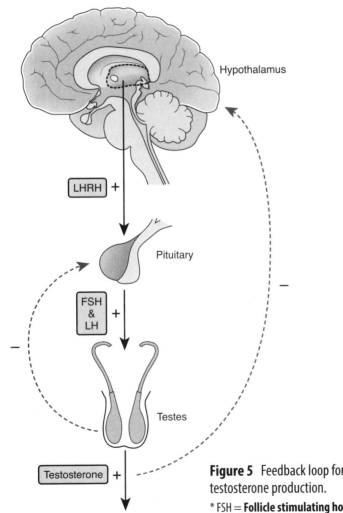

Figure 5 Feedback loop for testosterone production.
* FSH = **Follicle stimulating hormone**

Follicle stimulating hormone

A type of hormone produced by the pituitary that is involved in stimulating the production of sperm by the testicles.

stop producing LHRH, which in turn halts the production of testosterone by the testicles. It typically takes about 5 to 8 days for the LHRH agonists to drop testosterone levels significantly. LHRH agonists are given as shots which can be given monthly, every 3 months, every 4 months, every 6 months, or yearly, depending on your physician's choice.

An LHRH antagonist blocks the activity of LHRH, thus preventing it from stimulating the production of LH. As a result, the testicles are not stimulated to produce testosterone, which causes the testosterone levels to decrease. LHRH antagonists are not associated with an initial increase in testosterone and, in clinical trials, have been proven to rapidly decrease serum testosterone levels within 3 days. The currently approved LHRH antagonist is administered as a starting dose of two injections and then maintenance injections every 28 days.

Testicles

One of the two male reproductive organs that are located within the scrotum and produce testosterone and sperm.

Unlike a bilateral orchiectomy (the surgical removal of both **testicles**), which leads to a permanent change in the testosterone level, the effect of LHRH agonists and antagonists on serum testosterone is not permanent; thus, regular administration of the therapy is required.

4. My doctor wants to check my testosterone level to make sure it is a "castrate level." What is a castrate level of testosterone?

The majority of testosterone (about 95%) is produced by the testes and a small amount (about 5%) is produced by the adrenal glands. The serum testosterone level in young males varies throughout the day, often higher in the morning than later in the day. In older men, this variability is not as dramatic. There are no generally accepted normal testosterone levels related to age, and the definition of a "normal testosterone range" can vary from lab to lab. In general, a testosterone level between 400 ng/mL and 700 ng/mL is normal for a healthy, younger male. When production of testosterone by the testes is stopped, whether by bilateral orchiectomy or medical castration, the testosterone level will drop down to a "castrate" level. A castrate level of testosterone is defined as less than 20–50 ng/mL. Ten to twelve percent of the men treated with ADT, an LHRH agonist/antagonist alone or in combination with an **androgen receptor** blocker, fail to achieve castrate levels of testosterone. Since failure to lower the testosterone level to castrate levels can lead to the growth and spread of prostate cancer, it is important to ensure that the ADT is successful. If castrate testosterone levels are not achieved with ADT, your doctor might shorten the interval of injections, administering an LHRH injection every 3 months instead of 6 months, for instance, or recommend a bilateral orchiectomy.

The progression of prostate cancer due to ineffective ADT can be misdiagnosed as CRPC. As a result, it is essential to ensure that the testosterone level is at a castrate level before assuming that the prostate cancer is **castration resistant**.

5. If my cancer needs testosterone to grow, why is it growing when my testosterone level is "castrate"?

Although the treatment of advanced prostate cancer is focused on decreasing testosterone levels in order to slow prostate cancer growth, it is the androgen receptor (AR)

When production of testosterone by the testes is stopped, whether by bilateral orchiectomy or medical castration, the testosterone level will drop down to a "castrate" level.

Androgen receptor

A structure within the cell where androgen (testosterone and dihydrotestosterone [DHT]) binds and is translocated (moved) into the cell to stimulate cell growth through the production of various proteins.

Receptor

A protein molecule located in either the outer edge of the cell or the inside of the cell. When substances bind to it, they direct the cell to do something.

Castration resistant

Prostate cancer that progresses despite androgen deprivation therapy and resultant low (< 20–50 ng/dL) testosterone level.

Most castration-resistant prostate cancers remain sensitive to testosterone and adapt to be able to grow with the little testosterone available.

Dihydrotestos-terone (DHT)

A breakdown product of testosterone that is more potent than testosterone.

that is the main driver for the growth of prostate cancer cells. Either testosterone or a product of testosterone, **dihydrotestosterone (DHT)**, attaches to the AR in the prostate cancer cell. This androgen receptor with testosterone/DHT attached then moves into the center of the prostate cancer cell, the nucleus, where it can bind and influence the growth of the cancer. See **Figure 6**.

A variety of factors may allow the prostate cancer to grow despite testosterone being maintained at castrate level. Most castration-resistant prostate cancers remain

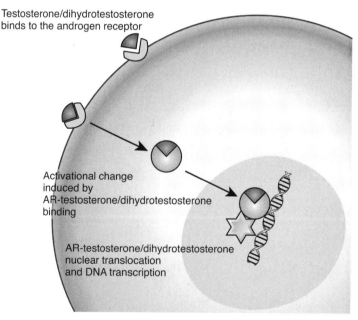

Figure 6 The interaction between testosterone/dihydrotestosterone and the androgen receptor.

sensitive to testosterone and adapt to be able to grow with the little testosterone available. The cancer can do this by increasing the number of androgen receptors on the **cell**, enabling each one to bind as much testosterone as possible. Additionally, the AR can adapt to allow other molecules to bind and stimulate the growth of the cancer cell. The cancer cells can become able to produce testosterone themselves or changes can occur in the genes and **enzymes** within the cell to magnify the response of the available testosterone on cell growth. Over time CRPC might evolve into a cancer that is androgen independent and thus be "hormone refractory."

Cell

The smallest unit of the body. Tissues in the body are made up of cells.

Enzyme

A chemical that is produced by living cells that causes chemical reactions to occur without undergoing any changes itself.

THE BASICS

13

PART TWO

Evaluation for Metastatic Castration-Resistant Prostate Cancer

How is mCRPC diagnosed?

My doctor recommended a bone, PET, or CT scan
to see if I have cancer in my bones. Why?

My doctor also recommended a
bone density scan. Why?

6. How is mCRPC diagnosed?

A PSA level that continues to rise even after definitive treatment (e.g., **radiation therapy**, radical **prostatectomy**, **brachytherapy**) is often the first sign of recurrent and/or metastatic prostate cancer. Up to 40% of men will eventually develop metastatic prostate cancer despite local treatment. However, some men, less than 5%, may present with extensive prostate cancer at the time of **diagnosis** and have **metastases** to the pelvic lymph nodes and/or bone metastases. In both situations, ADT, which is the use of LHRH agonists/antagonists to lower the testosterone level, will eventually be started. ADT is effective in decreasing the volume of prostate cancer and lowering the PSA level but is not curative. Typically, ADT is effective in shrinking the prostate cancer metastases/controlling the growth of the prostate cancer for about 2 to 3 years. However, changes within the prostate cancer cells allow those prostate cancer cells to adapt and grow despite very low levels of testosterone (see Question 5), referred to as castration-resistant prostate cancer (CRPC). When this occurs, the PSA level increases and metastases develop. The physician will periodically order **bone scans** and sometimes CT scans to check for the presence of radiographic metastases. Your doctor will also ask about signs and symptoms of metastatic disease, such as the onset of any bone pain and lower extremity swelling.

mCRPC is diagnosed when the presence of identifiable metastases (most commonly bone or lymph node metastases, rarely visible metastases) is found in a man with prostate cancer who is receiving ADT and has castrate levels of testosterone. About 90% of men with mCRPC have bone metastases, which is the only site of known **disease** in about 70% of men with mCRPC. The PSA level

Radiation therapy

Use of radioactive beams or implants to kill cancer cells.

Prostatectomy

The removal of the prostate gland and the tissue surrounding it.

Brachytherapy

A form of radiation therapy in which radioactive pellets are inserted inside of the prostate.

Diagnosis

The identification of the cause or presence of a medical problem or disease.

Metastases

See metastatic cancer.

Bone scan

A specialized nuclear medicine scan that allows doctors to detect changes in the bone that might be related to metastatic prostate cancer.

will rise in most men with the development of mCRPC. However, in rare instances of aggressive prostate cancer and hormone-refractory prostate cancer, metastases can develop without significant increases in PSA levels.

7. My doctor recommended a bone, PET, or CT scan to see if I have cancer in my bones. Why?

When the PSA level increases while a patient is on ADT, there is a concern about developing metastases. About 90% of men with mCRPC develop bone metastases. Bone metastases may cause pain and weaken the bone, increasing the **risk** of bone fracture. If you are asymptomatic with a rising PSA on ADT, your doctor will often start with a bone scan to determine if there are any areas that indicate possible bone metastases. A bone scan is a specialized nuclear scan that allows doctors to detect changes in the bone that could be related to metastatic prostate cancer. During the scan, a small amount of a radioactive chemical is injected through a vein into your bloodstream. This chemical then circulates through your body and is picked up by areas of fast bone growth, such as those that might be associated with cancer. The areas that pick up the radioactively labeled chemical will appear as dark spots on the bone scan (see Figure 1). Bone scans are the standard test to check for metastases in men with prostate cancer; however, limitations to the scan's **sensitivity** and **specificity** sometimes exist. Other conditions affecting the bones, such as a broken bone, arthritis, and a condition called Paget's disease, can cause an increase in uptake of the radioactive chemical, which can present difficulties in bone scan interpretation. By mimicking the appearance of metastatic disease in the bone scan, these conditions can potentially decrease the

Disease

Any change from or interruption of the normal structure or function of any part, organ, or system of the body that presents with characteristic symptoms and signs and whose cause and prognosis could be known or unknown.

Risk

The chance or probability that an adverse outcome will occur.

Sensitivity

The probability that a diagnostic test can correctly identify the presence of a particular disease.

Specificity

The probability that a diagnostic test can correctly identify the absence of disease.

X-ray

A type of high-energy radiation that can be used at low levels to make images of the internal structures of the body and at high levels for radiation therapy.

Computerized tomography/computerized axial tomography (CT/CAT) scan

A specialized X-ray study that allows doctors to visualize internal structures in cross-section to look for abnormalities.

Magnetic resonance imaging (MRI)

A study that is similar to a CT scan in that it allows one to see internal structures in detail, but different in that it does not involve radiation.

In a small number of men (8%), the bone scan can be normal when bone metastases are present.

specificity of a bone scan for bone metastases. Most of the time, though, correlation with the patient's history and additional radiologic studies such as a plain **X-ray**, **computerized tomography (CT)** scan, or **magnetic resonance imaging (MRI)** scan can minimize such confusion and determine with a relatively high degree of accuracy whether the abnormal area on the bone scan indicates the presence of cancer.

The bone scan is sensitive, but it does not identify small numbers of cancer cells in the bones and thus can miss very small areas of metastasis. In a small number of men (8%), the bone scan can be normal when bone metastases are present. A way to improve the sensitivity and specificity of a bone scan is to add **single photon emission computerized tomography (SPECT)** to the bone scan. During a SPECT scan, the camera rotates around the body, taking images as it rotates, as opposed to a regular bone scan, in which the camera passes straight over the body. The addition of SPECT allows one to see smaller areas in more detail.

Positron emission tomography (PET) scans using various radioactively labeled chemicals might be a more appropriate test for the detection of prostate cancer bone metastases, with studies showing improvements in the sensitivity and specificity of PET scans using ^{18}F and ^{11}C-labeled markers over regular bone scans. ^{18}**F-fluoride** and ^{11}C-choline PET scans have been approved by the **Food and Drug Administration (FDA)** for bone imaging. The PET scan produces three-dimensional color images of functional processes within the body. The PET scan involves the injection of a radioactive chemical that is attached (or tagged) to a natural chemical such as fluoride or choline. The tagged natural chemical is called a radiotracer. The radiotracer is injected into the body through a vein and circulates through the body, going to the organs that use the natural chemical. As the radiotracer is broken down in the body, positively charged particles called positrons are released, which in turn release energy. The energy appears as a three-dimensional (3-D) image on a computer monitor. These images are reviewed by a specialized doctor called a radiologist. ^{11}C-choline PET–CT can also be used to determine if there are lymph node metastases (see Figure 2) with a higher sensitivity than MRI or PET-only scanning and could prove useful in the future for detecting recurrent prostate cancer.

8. My doctor also recommended a bone density scan. Why?

A recent Gallup survey of American men revealed that most men believe that **osteoporosis** is "a women's disease." Osteoporosis is the loss of bone density, which leads to weakened bones that break more easily. Osteoporosis can affect men, particularly men receiving ADT. Risk factors for osteoporosis include:

- *Family history*: patients with a family history of decreased bone density are at an at least 50% increased risk of developing osteoporosis.

- *Increased age*: most men and women lose about 0.5% of bone mass every year after the age of 50.

- *Lifestyle*: decreased calcium and vitamin D intake, smoking, excessive alcohol consumption, caffeine intake, a lack of exercise, or immobilization.

- *Diseases associated with bone loss*: **chronic obstructive pulmonary disease (COPD)**, malabsorption syndrome, hyperparathyroidism, **hypogonadism**, renal insufficiency, and vitamin D deficiency.

Single photon emission computerized tomography (SPECT)

A type of nuclear imaging test that uses a radioactive substance and a special camera to create three-dimensional pictures.

Positron emission tomography (PET)

A nuclear imaging technique that produces a three-dimensional image or picture of a functional process in the body.

Food and Drug Administration (FDA)

The federal agency responsible for the approval of prescription medications in the United States.

Osteoporosis

Reduction in the amount of bone mass, leading to fractures after minimal trauma.

Lifestyle

The way a person chooses to live.

Chronic obstructive pulmonary disease (COPD)

A group of lung diseases that block airflow and make breathing difficult.

Hypogonadism

In males, a condition in which the testicles do not produce enough testosterone.

Dual energy X-ray absorptiometry (DEXA) scan

An imaging system to assess bone mineral density.

Noninvasive

Not requiring any incision or the insertion of an instrument or substance into the body.

Low testosterone levels affect bone mineral density in men almost the same as low estrogen levels in women.

• *Medications*: such as immunosuppressive medications, anti-seizure medications, or glucocorticoid medications (steroid medications used to treat diseases such as asthma and rheumatoid arthritis).

How can you tell if osteoporosis is occurring? The best way to check your bone mineral density is with a **dual energy X-ray absorptiometry (DEXA) scan,** the same study used to evaluate for osteoporosis in women. It is a **noninvasive** (meaning it does not require an incision or the insertion of an instrument or substance into the body), precise, and quick test that involves minimal radiation exposure. The test measures the bone mineral density, which is compared to values obtained from healthy young adult control subjects. The controls have been well established for women but are less clear for men. In addition, there appears to be an ethnic variability in bone density, with African American males usually having higher peak bone mass and a lower risk of osteoporotic fractures than white males. Normally, the bone mineral density is at its highest by age 25 and begins to decline after age 35, with both men and women losing 0.3% to 0.5% of their bone mass per year as part of the normal aging process. Men have a higher peak bone mass than women.

Several factors contribute to loss of bone mineral density, but decreased sex hormone production (i.e., testosterone, estrogen) has the most significant impact on bone mineral density. Low testosterone levels affect bone mineral density in men almost the same as low estrogen levels in women. The use of androgen deprivation therapy, whether it is via orchiectomy or LHRH agonist/antagonist with or without anti-androgen, causes decreased bone mineral density. There is an average loss of 4% per year for the first 2 years on ADT (**hormone therapy**) and 2% per year after year 4, which is similar to the loss in women after removal of the ovaries or natural menopause. This loss of bone mineral density in men on ADT occurs for at least 10 years and probably accounts for the increased incidence of fractures: 5% to 13.5% of men taking hormone therapy have fractures, compared to 1% in men with prostate cancer who are not on ADT. LHRH agonists/antagonists appear to increase the risk of clinical fractures, and treatment duration correlates with fracture risk.

Men with prostate cancer being treated with ADT are often prescribed calcium and vitamin D to help prevent bone loss. However, bone loss can still occur despite taking vitamin D and calcium. Thus, it is important to have a bone scan obtained periodically to determine if you are developing osteoporosis so that it can be treated (see Question 16).

Hormone therapy

The manipulation of a disease's natural history and symptoms through the use of hormones.

PART THREE

Treatment of Metastatic Castration-Resistant Prostate Cancer

I am on a "maximum androgen blockade" pill (androgen receptor blocker) and am receiving LHRH agonist/antagonist shots. My doctor wants me to stop the pill. Will this lower my PSA and, if so, for how long?

My doctor wants me to try another form of therapy for my mCRPC but recommends that I also continue receiving hormone therapy shots. Why do I need to continue the shots if they are not working?

My doctor says that now there are several treatment options available to treat mCRPC. What are they? What happens if my mCRPC continues to grow on one of these therapies? Can I try another?

More…

9. I am on a "maximum androgen blockade" pill (androgen receptor blocker) and am receiving LHRH agonist/antagonist shots. My doctor wants me to stop the pill. Will this lower my PSA and, if so, for how long?

American Urological Association (AUA)

A professional association in the United States for urologists.

Total (maximal) androgen blockade

The total blockage of production and action of testosterone through surgery and/or medications.

In individuals with non-metastatic CRPC who are unwilling to undergo observation, the LHRH agonist/antagonist is continued, and another medication, an anti-androgen, can be added.

LHRH agonists/antagonists are the first-line treatment for men with advanced prostate cancer (increasing PSA after radical prostatectomy, radiation therapy, brachytherapy, or those initially presenting with metastatic prostate cancer without prior therapy) and those who present with metastatic disease at the time of diagnosis. LHRH agonists/antagonists are very effective at lowering PSA levels and slowing down the growth of prostate cancer. They do not, however, cure you of prostate cancer, and, over time, the prostate cancer will adapt to the low testosterone levels and continue to progress. When your PSA levels increase while you are on LHRH agonist/antagonist therapy, your doctor may check your serum testosterone level to make sure that the LHRH agonist/antagonist is dropping the testosterone to almost undetectable levels (< 20–50 ng/dL). If the testosterone level is low on LHRH agonist/antagonist therapy and your PSA level is still increasing, you have CRPC. In the absence of metastases, the **American Urological Association (AUA)** recommends observation with continued ADT. However, in individuals with nonmetastatic CRPC who are unwilling to undergo observation, the LHRH agonist/antagonist is continued, and another medication, an anti-androgen, can be added. This combined therapy is called **total (maximal) androgen blockade** and is often effective in treating the prostate cancer for 3 to 6 months. Anti-androgens are androgen receptor blockers that prevent the attachment of androgens (testosterone and DHT) to the AR, thus preventing the stimulus for the growth of the cancer cells. Thus, total (maximal) androgen blockade effectively decreases the amount of testosterone in the body and prevents the testosterone that is being produced from acting on the prostate cancer cells. At some point in time, the prostate cancer will progress despite **maximum androgen blockade** and PSA levels will start to go up again. If maximal androgen blockade fails, some men (up to 30%) benefit from withdrawal (stopping) of the anti-androgen, showing clinical improvement and decreased PSA levels. Individuals who respond in this manner can expect about 6 months of improved **quality of life**.

Dihydrotestosterone (DHT)

A breakdown product of testosterone that is more potent than testosterone.

Maximum androgen blockade

The combination of androgen deprivation therapy and an androgen receptor blocker.

Quality of life

An evaluation of healthy status relative to the patient's age, expectations, and physical and mental capabilities.

10. My doctor wants me to try another form of therapy for my mCRPC, but recommends that I also continue receiving hormone therapy shots. Why do I need to continue the shots if they are not working?

The cancer cells in most men who have CRPC and mCRPC are not **refractory**. However, over time they adapt to low levels of testosterone by learning to maximally utilize the little testosterone that is available and to make their own testosterone and DHT. Prostate cancer cell growth is controlled by the number of testosterone/DHT-AR complexes there are present. One way the prostate cancer cells can adapt to the low level of testosterone is to increase the number of available AR to increase the likelihood that enough androgen-AR complexes will form to stimulate prostate cancer cell growth. Additional changes in the AR may allow it to

Refractory

Resistant to therapy.

bind to the androgen more tightly and allow it to move into the nucleus more efficiently, increasing the likelihood of a response to the available testosterone. This continued "sensitivity" to androgens is why your doctor recommends that you continue the ADT in addition to trying another form of therapy for your mCRPC. This understanding of the continued role of the AR has led to the development of new therapies aimed at further decreasing androgen production or blocking the function of the AR.

11. My doctor says that now there are several treatment options available to treat mCRPC. What are they? What happens if my CRPC continues to grow on one of these therapies? Can I try another?

Indications

The reasons for undertaking a specific treatment, such as choice of therapy, surgical, medical, or other.

Side effect

A reaction to a medication or treatment.

Performance status

In medicine (oncology and other fields), performance status is an attempt to quantify cancer patients' general well-being and activities of daily life. There are two commonly used scoring systems: the Karnofsky and the ECOG/WHO/Zubrod.

Prednisone

A synthetic drug similar to corticosterone.

There are several new therapies for the treatment of mCRPC. These therapies differ in the **indications** for their use, the way they are given, the way that they act, and their **side effects** (see **Table 1**). Thus, it is important that you understand these differences as you choose the next step in treatment of your prostate cancer. The different therapies can be divided into those that affect the production of testosterone, those that affect the AR, chemotherapies that affect the growth of the prostate cancer cells, and immunotherapies that help your immune system fight off the prostate cancer cells. The choice between these therapies may depend on whether or not you have symptoms of metastatic prostate cancer, your overall **performance status**, and what therapies you have tried in the past. There is also a new therapy to help decrease the risk of bone complications from metastasis

26

Table 1 Treatments

Therapy and Approved Indication	Dosing	Effect on Overall Survival	Other Effects	Side Effects
First-line chemotherapy: taxane *Indication: CRPC and mCRPC*	Intravenous over 60 minutes every 3 weeks plus **prednisone**	19.2 months compared to 16.3 with an older form of **chemotherapy**	Reduction in pain, rates of PSA level response higher, and better quality of life than older form of chemotherapy	*Contraindication:* prior hypersensitivity to taxane or polysorbate, neutrophil count < 1,500 cells/mm^3 *Warning/Caution:* may affect heart conduction and rarely require pacemaker placement, use with caution with concomitant use of medications that affect the CYP2C8 and CYP3A4 enzymes, hypersensitivity reactions may occur resulting in shortness of breath, low blood pressure, angioedema and urticaria, may cause liver toxicity, fluid retention and toxic death *Side effects:* neutropenia, fatigue, alopecia, nausea/vomiting, diarrhea, nail changes, **sensory neuropathy**, changes in taste, **stomatitis**, abnormal liver function tests
Second-line chemotherapy: taxane *Indication: mCRPC recfractory to first-line taxane*	Intravenous over 60 minutes every 3 weeks plus prednisone	15.1 months compared to 12.7 months for older form of chemotherapy	Significantly better **progression-free survival**, decrease in tumor, and decrease in PSA level	*Contraindication:* prior hypersensitivity to taxane or polysorbate, neutrophil count < 1,500 cells/mm^3 *Warning/Caution:* may affect heart conduction and rarely require pacemaker placement, use with caution with concomitant use of medications that affect the CYP2C8 and CYP3A4 enzymes, hypersensitivity reactions may occur resulting in shortness of breath, low blood pressure, angioedema and urticaria, may cause liver toxicity, fluid retention and toxic death. Caution regarding use in patients with elevated bilirubin *Side effects:* neutropenia, fatigue, alopecia, nausea/vomiting, diarrhea, nail changes, sensory neuropathy, changes in taste, stomatitis, abnormal liver function tests, **thrombocytopenia**

(continued)

Taxane(s)

A chemotherapy drug derived from the Yew plant that prevents cell growth by inhibiting special cell structures, called microtubules, which are involved in cell division.

Chemotherapy

A treatment for cancer that uses powerful chemicals to weaken and destroy the cancer cells.

Alopecia

Partial or complete loss of hair from parts of the body where it normally grows (baldness).

Sensory neuropathy

Damage to the nerves of the peripheral nervous system that can cause abnormal sensations, like tingling or a prick-like feeling.

Stomatitis

Inflammation of the lining of the mouth.

Progression-free survival

The length of time during and after medication or treatment during which the disease being treated (cancer) does not get worse.

Thrombocytopenia

A decrease in the platelet count of the blood.

Hypokalemia

Lower-than-normal potassium levels due to excessive excretion or inadequate uptake at the cellular level.

Table 1 Treatments (continued)

Therapy and Approved Indication	Dosing	Effect on Overall Survival	Other Effects	Side Effects
Immunotherapy *Indication: asymptomatic or minimally symptomatic mCRPC*	Each cycle involves removal of blood, harvesting and activation of specialized immune cells, and reinfusion. A complete course is 3 cycles, each cycle separated by 2 weeks	3.7 to 4.5 months for immunotherapy compared to placebo	Time to progression of the cancer was 0.2 weeks to 2.6 weeks longer with immunotherapy than placebo. There was no significant difference in reduction of PSA by at least 50% between immunotherapy and placebo	Most common side effects include chills, fever, fatigue, nausea, joint ache, and headache, which usually occur within first few days of treatment
CYP17 inhibitor (inhibitor of androgen production by testes, adrenal glands, and prostate cancer cells) *Indication: mCRPC*	Four 250 mg tablets orally once a day, on an empty stomach, plus prednisone 5 mg orally twice a day	15.8 months compared to 11.2 months for placebo in patients who had received prior chemotherapy containing docetaxel; in patients with mCRPC who did not receive prior chemotherapy, 35.3 months compared to 30.1 months with placebo plus prednisone	Significantly increased median radiographic progression-free survival was noted with CYP17 inhibitor compared to placebo plus prednisone in patients with mCRPC who did not receive prior chemotherapy. Significant delayed median time to chemotherapy and significantly delayed median time to opiate use in patients with mCRPC who did not receive prior chemotherapy	*Warning/Caution:* Use with caution in patients with heart disease; monitor for signs and symptoms of adrenal insufficiency; may need to increase doses of prednisone during stressful situations; may cause hypertension, **hypokalemia**, and edema; control hypertension and correct hypokalemia before treatment; monitor liver function for signs of liver toxicity; should not be used in patients with severe liver impairment; may be affected by concomitant use of other medications that affect CYP3A4 and CYP2D6 enzymes. *Side effects:* fatigue, joint swelling or discomfort, edema, hot flushes, diarrhea, vomiting, cough, shortness of breath, urinary tract infection, bruising, hypertension, hypokalemia, high blood sugar, high cholesterol, abnormal liver function tests, hypophosphatemia, muscle discomfort

Therapy and Approved Indication	Dosing	Effect on Overall Survival	Other Effects	Side Effects
Androgen Receptor Inhibitor *Indication: mCRPC with previous trial of first-line chemotherapy*	Four 40 mg (160 mg) capsules once a day, with or without food	18.4 months compared to 13.6 months with placebo in patients with mCRPC after first-line chemotherapy	Greater percentage of patients with PSA decrease of 50% or more, better reduction in soft tissue metastases, better quality of life with androgen receptor inhibitor compared to placebo in patients with mCRPC after first-line chemotherapy Time to PSA progression 8.3 months versus 3.0 months with placebo Time to first skeletal-related adverse event 16.7 months compared to 13.3 months with placebo in patients with mCRPC with prior trial of first-line chemotherapy	*Warning/Caution:* may be affected by concomitant use of medications that affect CYP2C8, CYP3A4, CYP2C9, and CYP2C19 enzymes. Has not been studied in patients with history of seizures *Side effects:* **asthenia**, fatigue, back pain, diarrhea, arthralgia, hot flush, edema of lower extremities, muscle pain, headache, **upper and lower respiratory tract infections**, muscle weakness, dizziness, insomnia, spinal cord compression, blood in the urine, **paresthesia**, anxiety, high blood pressure, seizure
Radionuclide therapy *Symptomatic mCRPC with bone metastases without visceral metastases*	50 kBq per kg/body weight given at 4 week intervals for 6 injections	14.9 months for radionuclide compared to 11.3 months for placebo	Time to first symptomatic skeletal event significantly longer with radionuclide therapy, 15.6 months compared to 9.8 months for placebo	*Warning/Caution:* therapy can cause significant bone marrow suppression—measure blood counts before starting therapy and before each treatment *Side effects:* nausea, diarrhea, vomiting, peripheral edema, anemia, low white blood cell count, low platelet count

Please refer to the full Prescribing Information provided by the drug manufacturer for complete information on a particular drug, including a complete list of side effects and warnings/precautions.

Asthenia
Abnormal physical weakness or lack of energy.

Arthralgia
Joint pain.

Edema
Swelling caused by excess fluid trapped in the body's tissue.

Upper respiratory tract infection
An acute infection involving the nose, sinuses, and throat.

Lower respiratory tract infection
Acute infection involving bronchi (bronchitis) and/or lungs (pneumonia).

Paresthesia
Abnormal sensation, typically tingling or pricking, that could be due to nerve damage.

CYP17 inhibitor
An inhibitor of an enzyme found in steroid-hormone-producing tissues, adrenal glands, testicles, and prostate cancer cells.

to the bones. Establishing a performance status is an attempt to quantify cancer patients' general well-being and activities of daily life. It is often used to determine if an individual is healthy enough to receive chemotherapy and if the dose needs to be modified. There are two commonly used scoring systems: the Karnofsky and the ECOG/WHO/Zubrod (see **Table 2**).

To help patients make treatment choice decisions, the AUA has recently published a guide on CRPC (*www.auanet.org*). Management recommendations are based on the presence/absence of symptoms, the patient's performance status, and any prior therapy. The guide identifies standard treatment regimens and alternative therapies. The National Comprehensive Cancer Network (NCCN) also has guidelines available for patients (*www.nccn.org/patients/guidelines/prostate/index.html*).

First-line treatments for mCRPC include:
- Continuation of androgen deprivation therapy and observation if the patient is asymptomatic
- Immunotherapy—if the patient is asymptomatic or minimally symptomatic
- CYP17 inhibitor plus prednisone
- First-line taxane chemotherapy
- Radionuclide therapy may be used if patient has symptomatic bone metastases without visceral metastases

For patients who have been treated with prior first-line taxane therapy the treatment options include:
- CYP17 inhibitor plus prednisone
- Second-line taxane chemotherapy
- Newer androgen receptor blocker

Table 2 Performance Scoring Systems

Karnofsky Scoring (score ranges from 100–0)		ECOG/WHO/Zubrod (score ranges from 0 to 5)	
100%	normal, no complaints, no signs of disease	0	asymptomatic—fully active, no restrictions
90%	able to carry out normal activity, few symptoms or signs of disease	1	symptomatic, but completely ambulatory, able to carry out light work
80%	normal activity with some difficulty, some symptoms or signs	2	symptomatic, < 50% time in bed during the day— ambulatory but unable to carry out any work activities— can care for self
70%	able to care for self, but not capable of normal activity or work	3	symptomatic, > 50% time in bed during the day, limited ability to care for self
60%	requiring some help, can take care of most personal care	4	bedbound—completely disabled, cannot care for self
50%	often needs help, frequent need for medical care	5	death
40%	disabled, requires special care and assistance		
30%	severely disabled, hospitalization indicated but not at risk of death		
20%	very ill, urgent admission required, needs supportive measures or treatment		
10%	terminal, rapidly progressive fatal disease processes		
0%	death		

Data from: Karnofsky performance score - Karnofsky DA, Burchenal JH. (1949) The clinical evaluation of chemotherapeutic agents in cancer. In: MacLeod (CM) (ed). *Evaluation of chemotherapeutic Agents*. Columbia University Press. p. 196; ECOG/WHO/Zubrod - Oken MM, Creech RH, Tormey DC, et al. (1982) Toxicity and response criteria of the Eastern Cooperative Oncology Group. *Am J Clin Oncol 5*(6): 649-655.

Immunotherapy

Treatment of disease by inducing, enhancing, or suppressing an immune response.

Immune system

A complex group of organs, tissues, blood cells, and substances that work to fight off infections, cancers, or foreign substances.

Prostatic acid phosphatase

An antigen produced by the prostate.

Antigen-presenting cell (APC)

A cell (dendritic cell) that activates the immune system by processing and presenting antigen to specialized immune cells (T cells) to activate them to reject and destroy cancer cells.

A complete course of immunotherapy involves completing this process three times, with 2 weeks in between each time.

- Re-treatment with first-line taxane chemotherapy if the discontinuation was due to reversible side effects and the patient demonstrated a response to treatment with the first-line taxane chemotherapy
- Radionuclide therapy if the patient has symptomatic bone metastases without visceral metastases

Your doctor may recommend a certain therapy for you based on your performance status, your other medical problems, and other medications.

12. What is immunotherapy for mCRPC? What are the side effects?

Immunotherapy is the prevention or treatment of disease with substances that stimulate the **immune system**. The goal of immunotherapy is to stimulate the immune system to reject and destroy cancer cells. Cancer cells that produce antigens are optimal targets for immunotherapy. Prostate cancer is one of these cancers, as the majority of prostate cancer cells produce two antigens: PSA and **prostatic acid phosphatase.**

The immunotherapy used for prostate cancer involves a three-step process. The first step is taking a blood sample to collect specialized white blood cells, called **antigen-presenting cells (APCs),** or **dendritic cells**, from the blood. These cells are then mixed with a special protein called a **fusion protein**. The fusion protein has two parts to it: the antigen prostatic acid phosphatase, which is found in the majority of prostate cancer cells, and **granulocyte-macrophage colony-stimulating factor (GM-CSF),** which causes these APCs to mature. The mature APCs are then re-infused into your body, where they activate specialized cells in your body's immune system called T cells, which reject and destroy cells that have prostatic acid phosphatase antigen (see **Figure 7**). A complete course of the immunotherapy involves completing this process three times, with 2 weeks in between each time.

Currently, immunotherapy is approved for men with asymptomatic or minimally symptomatic mCRPC. Studies have demonstrated that immunotherapy increases overall survival 3.7–4.5 months longer than placebo treatment. The most common side effects of the therapy include chills, fever, fatigue, nausea, and headache; these typically occur within the first few days of treatment (see Table 1).

Dendritic cells

See antigen-presenting cells.

Fusion protein

A protein created by joining two or more genes responsible for the production of separate individual proteins, resulting in a protein that has functional properties derived from each of the original proteins.

Granulocyte-macrophage colony-stimulating factor (GM-CSF)

A protein secreted by several cells that stimulates the growth and development of various cells.

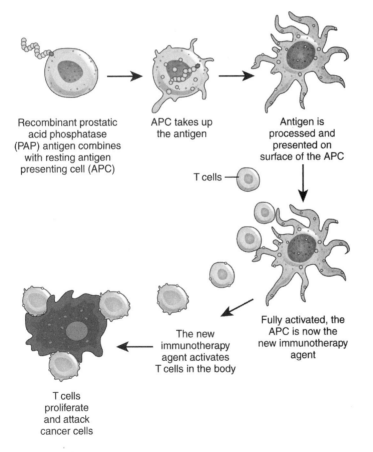

Recombinant prostatic acid phosphatase (PAP) antigen combines with resting antigen presenting cell (APC)

APC takes up the antigen

Antigen is processed and presented on surface of the APC

T cells

Fully activated, the APC is now the new immunotherapy agent

The new immunotherapy agent activates T cells in the body

T cells proliferate and attack cancer cells

Figure 7 Mechanism of action of immunotherapy.

13. What are therapies that target the androgen receptor? What are their side effects?

Androgen receptor blockers have been used for some time in men with an increasing PSA on ADT as part of maximal androgen blockade. This combination therapy has been shown to be effective in slowing down the growth of prostate cancer and increasing overall survival by about 3% to 5% at 5 years compared to monotherapy with an LHRH agonist/antagonist. However, the cancer cells eventually develop the ability to grow despite maximal androgen blockade. In the development of CRPC, there appear to be several changes that occur with the androgen receptor. First, there is an increase in the number of androgen receptors, enhancing the maximal binding of what little testosterone is available; second, they appear to bind to testosterone more tightly, increasing the chance that the testosterone-androgen receptor complex will be moved into the nucleus of the cell and stimulate the production of chemicals essential for cell growth. In addition, changes in the structure of the androgen receptor may lead to the older forms of androgen receptor blockers acting as a stimulant. It is thought that this combination of increased number of androgen receptors, tighter binding of androgen to the androgen receptor, and enhanced movement into the nucleus of the cell results in a 10,000-fold decrease in the amount of testosterone needed for cancer cell growth.

A new AR blocker has recently been approved by the FDA that differs from the older forms (see Table 1). The newer AR blocker binds tightly to the AR, preventing the binding of testosterone or DHT from moving into the nucleus of the cell, and from binding to DNA. As a result, the chemicals needed for cell growth are prevented from being produced (see **Figure 8**). Thus, the new androgen receptor blocker has three ways that it prevents the growth of prostate cancer cells and it does not act as a stimulant over time. Currently, this newer form of AR blocker is only approved for the treatment of mCRPC in patients for whom chemotherapy has been ineffective. However, ongoing studies are evaluating the role of this AR blocker in mCRPC patients for whom ADT has not been effective but who have not received chemotherapy. Studies are also comparing it to the older AR blockers to determine its use in maximal androgen blockade. The results of these studies may lead to the use of this new AR blocker in earlier stages of prostate cancer.

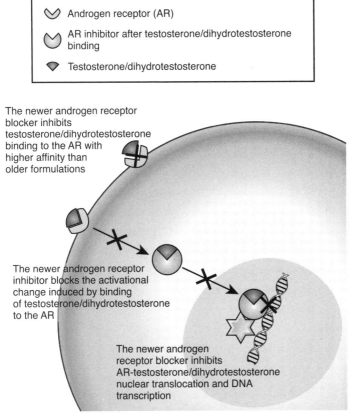

The newer androgen receptor blocker inhibits testosterone/dihydrotestosterone binding to the AR with higher affinity than older formulations

The newer androgen receptor inhibitor blocks the activational change induced by binding of testosterone/dihydrotestosterone to the AR

The newer androgen receptor blocker inhibits AR-testosterone/dihydrotestosterone nuclear translocation and DNA transcription

Androgen receptor (AR)

AR inhibitor after testosterone/dihydrotestosterone binding

Testosterone/dihydrotestosterone

Figure 8 Mechanism of action of the newer androgen receptor blocker.

14. Is chemotherapy used for mCRPC? What are the side effects?

Chemotherapy refers to the use of powerful drugs to either kill cancer cells or interfere with their growth. Many different types of chemotherapeutic agents work at different times in the growth cycle of the cell, and combinations of chemotherapeutic agents are often used to maximize the effect on cancer cells. Several different drugs have been shown to improve symptoms and decrease the PSA level or the amount of prostate cancer cells, though no drug has been shown to kill all of the cancer cells present. Ongoing **clinical trials** continue to look at new chemotherapy drugs, combinations of drugs, or different doses in hopes of finding more effective and less toxic options. Prior to the use of taxanes, several different types of chemotherapy drugs were used. Currently, taxanes are the most commonly used chemotherapy drug, both as first-line and second-line chemotherapy for mCRPC (see Table 1).

Taxanes are drugs that are derived from the Yew tree. They affect the growth of the prostate cancer cells by affecting their microtubules, preventing them from dividing. They have been shown to improve survival in men with mCRPC. One study demonstrated superior improvement in survival and quality of life and better pain control in men treated with a taxane compared to an alternative chemotherapy. A second-line taxane drug has been approved to treat mCRPC patients for whom first-line taxane is ineffective. This second-line taxane has been shown to be superior to an alternative chemotherapy drug.

Taxanes are administered intravenously, often in combination with a steroid, prednisone, to decrease their side effects. Side effects of the taxanes include fluid retention,

Clinical trial

A carefully planned and regulated experiment to evaluate a treatment or medication (often a new drug) for an unproven use.

dry skin, thickened and discolored nails, weight gain, and decreased blood cell production. Taxanes are prescribed by an **oncologist**, a medical specialist who is trained to evaluate and treat cancer.

Oncologist
A medical specialist who is trained to evaluate and treat cancer.

15. My doctor says that there are therapies that can stop testosterone production by other tissues in my body, even the prostate cancer itself. Is this true?

The testicles produce the majority of testosterone and testosterone precursors. However, the adrenal glands also produce a small amount of testosterone and testosterone precursors. In addition, prostate cancer cells can adapt to be able to produce testosterone themselves. The more commonly used ADTs (LHRH agonists/antagonists) affect only the production of testosterone produced by the testicles. As the prostate cancer cells become castrate resistant, they remain sensitive to testosterone, but adapt to lower testosterone levels and develop the ability to produce testosterone themselves. Therapies that can block testosterone production in both the adrenal glands and the prostate cancer cells have been shown to slow down the growth of prostate cancer. One such therapy that has recently been approved blocks the enzyme CYP17 (17 alpha-hydroxylase/C17,20 lyase), which is found in the testicular, adrenal, and prostate tissues and is required for testosterone production (see **Figure 9**). It also prevents the production of two important precursors of testosterone, dehydroepiandrosterone (DHEA) and androstenedione (see Figure 8). This therapy is useful in men for whom the more commonly used ADT has proven ineffective, as ADT affects only the production of testosterone in

Therapies that can block testosterone production in both the adrenal glands and the prostate cancer cells have been shown to slow down the growth of prostate cancer.

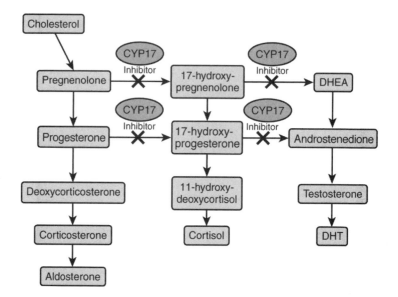

Figure 9 Mechanism of action of CYP17 inhibitor.

the testes and not the testosterone produced by the prostate cancer cells or the adrenal glands.

Androgens

Hormones that are necessary for the development and function of the male sexual organs and male sexual characteristics (hair, voice change). Testosterone and DHT are two types.

The adrenal gland is responsible for the production of three types of chemicals: **androgens** (DHEA, androstenedione, testosterone, and DHT), glucocorticoids (cortisol), and mineralocorticoids (corticosterone and aldosterone). In addition to affecting the production of androgens, CYP17 also decreases cortisol production and increases production of corticosterone and aldosterone (see Figure 9). The side effects of the therapy reflect these changes (see Table 1). Excess mineralocorticoids (corticosterone and aldosterone) can cause fluid retention, high blood pressure, and a drop in the body's potassium level. In some patients with a history of cardiovascular disease or heart failure, their heart condition may become worse. Taking prednisone, a synthetic chemical similar to corticosterone, can help decrease production of mineralocorticoids and these side effects (see Table 1).

16. What treatment options are available to prevent bone problems if I have weak bones from my hormone therapy?

Osteoporosis is common in both men and women. In fact, about 2 million men in the United States are at risk for osteoporosis and about one-third of all hip fractures are experienced by men. Question 8 addresses some of the general factors that increase the risk of osteoporosis in men. Men with prostate cancer who are on ADT are at risk for significant decreases in bone mineral density, with a decrease of 2% to 3% of bone mineral density per year in the hip and spine during initial therapy and a steady decline with long-term therapy. Several large studies suggest that this decline in bone mineral density increases the risk of clinical fractures. In addition to the effects of the ADT on bone mineral density, other factors that may increase the risk of clinical fractures in men on ADT include an increased risk of falling in men with metastatic disease and increased risk of treatment-related frailty.

About 2 million men in the United States are at risk for osteoporosis and about one-third of all hip fractures are experienced by men.

Several therapies are available for prevention and treatment of decreased bone mineral density in men on ADT:

- *Calcium and vitamin D*: Calcium and vitamin D supplementation is recommended in men on ADT to help prevent bone loss. However, in most men receiving ADT, calcium and vitamin D alone are not sufficient in preventing bone loss. The recommended dose of each is 400 IU/day for vitamin D and 1200–1500 mg/day for calcium.

- *Bisphosphonates*: **Bisphosphonates** are commonly used in women with osteoporosis. One bisphosphonate has been approved by the Food and Drug Administration for the prevention of skeletal complications in men with bone metastases from prostate cancer. It has been shown to decrease the risk of skeletal-related events in men with CRPC. It is an **intravenous** infusion that takes about 15 minutes and is given every 3 to 4 weeks. Because it should not be given if you are experiencing kidney problems, you will be given a blood test prior to each infusion. It is recommended that you continue your calcium and vitamin D supplementation in addition to the infusions. Side effects include nausea, fatigue, **anemia**, bone pain, constipation, fever, vomiting, and shortness of breath. A less common side effect of bisphosphonate is **osteonecrosis of the jaw (ONJ)**. ONJ is an uncommon but severe side effect of bisphosphonate. It can occur following dental surgery, such as after having a tooth removed. A sign of ONJ is poor healing of an area of bone exposed after dental surgery. There might or might not be pain, swelling, infection, or drainage associated with ONJ. Treatment of ONJ varies with severity. Unhealthy bone may need to be removed, and any associated infections should be treated. Rinsing your mouth with antibacterial mouth rinses helps prevent infections, and treatment with bisphosphonate should be stopped. There appears to be some improvement in ONJ at least 6 months after stopping treatment with the bisphosphonate.

Because of these potential complications, it is recommended that patients maintain good mouth hygiene and should have a dental examination with preventive dentistry prior to starting bisphosphonate. You should also inform your dentist before starting a bisphosphonate so that any necessary dental procedures can be performed before your bisphosphonate treatment starts. Ideally you should avoid any invasive dental procedures while on a bisphosphonate. If you need an invasive dental procedure while taking a bisphosphonate, it is unclear whether stopping the bisphosphonate decreases the risk of ONJ.

- *RANK-ligand (RANKL) inhibitor*: Our bones are continuously being remodeled. Old bone tissue is removed and replaced with new bone tissue. There are specialized cells called **osteoblasts** that make new bones and cells called **osteoclasts** that break down bone. The body doesn't make osteoclasts directly, however. Rather, there are cells called **pre-osteoclasts** that are stimulated to develop into osteoclasts when a special molecule, the **cytokine** RANKL, attaches to a RANKL receptor on the cell. An **antibody** has been developed that prevents RANKL from attaching to the pre-osteoclast, thus the stimulation required for the pre-osteoclast to develop into an osteoclast is blocked, preventing the breakdown of bone (see **Figure 10**). A study was performed in which 1,468 prostate cancer patients receiving ADT and vitamin D and calcium were randomized to receive either a RANKL inhibitor or a placebo every 6 months for 36 months. The results demonstrated a lower incidence of bone fractures in those men taking the RANKL inhibitor (1.5%) than in those taking a placebo (3.9%).

The most common side effects of treatment with the RANKL inhibitor include urinary tract infection (e.g., bladder infection) and lower respiratory tract infection (e.g., lung infection), cataracts, constipation, rashes, eczema, and joint pain. The RANKL

RANK-ligand (RANKL)

A cytokine involved in the development of osteoclasts from pre-osteoclasts.

Osteoblast

A specialized cell that makes new bone.

Osteoclast

A specialized cell that breaks down bone.

Pre-osteoclast

A specialized cell that develops into an osteoclast when stimulated by RANK-ligand.

Cytokine

Any of a number of substances secreted by certain cells of the immune system that regulate responses to infection, immune responses, inflammation, and trauma.

Antibody

A molecule produced by the body that reacts with a specific antigen that induced its synthesis.

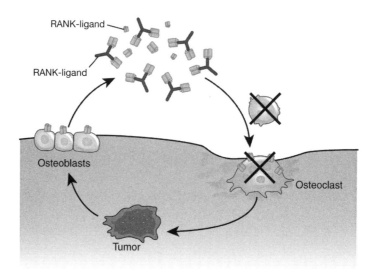

Figure 10 Mechanism of action of RANKL inhibitors.

inhibitor should not be used if the calcium level in the bloodstream is low (known as **hypocalcemia**). Thus, it is important to take vitamin D and calcium supplements while on a RANKL inhibitor and to have your calcium levels checked before starting treatment. As with the bisphosphonates, the RANKL inhibitor could increase the risk of ONJ following removal of teeth or other oral surgery. Similar dental precautions should be taken with the RANKL inhibitor as with the bisphosphonates.

17. What treatment options are available if I have cancer in my bones?

Most patients with advanced prostate cancer will have painful bone metastases during the course of their disease. The use of ADT results in improvement in pain in most men with bone metastases. However, in patients with mCRPC, the pain from bone metastases is often a recurrent problem. The newer therapies for treating mCRPC can also help with painful bone metastases. Radiation therapy directed at specific bones can be useful for treating isolated bone metastases.

For men with more significant pain and more extensive bone metastases, intravenous radionuclide treatments that are directed to bone metastases can be helpful. The FDA has approved several agents. When injected intravenously, they are preferentially taken up by the tumorous bone and "radiate" the bone. Because the bone marrow produces blood cells, a drop in the white blood cell count (the cell that helps fight off infections) and **platelet** count (the cell which helps form blood clots) are the most common adverse effects of these agents. Because your kidneys will get rid of the radionuclide by excreting it in the urine, your doctor will want to run a blood test to make sure your kidneys are working adequately prior to administering the radionuclide. The overall response rate to the treatment ranges from 33% to 82%, with complete pain resolution reported in 8% to 77% of men treated, and 15% to 50% of men experience a reduction in pain. In addition to its effects on bones, the median overall survival was increased by 3.6 months with this therapy. Patients with a higher red blood cell count, less extensive bone metastases, a lower PSA level, and a better performance status appear to have a better response. Retreatment is possible with these agents; however, sufficient time must be given to allow for white blood cell and platelet counts to return to normal in between treatments. Prior chemotherapy does not appear to affect the results of these agents. Although radionuclide therapy can be used in conjunction with chemotherapy, there is the risk of significant lowering of the blood counts, increasing the risk of infection.

Radiation therapy directed at specific bones can be useful for treating isolated bone metastases.

Platelet
A cell found in large numbers in blood and involved in clotting.

Following the injection, the agents are excreted in the urine over the course of about 2 weeks. You should be very careful during this period. Avoid soiling undergarments or around toilet areas if possible, and sit down to urinate, as this minimizes the scatter of urine. After voiding, be sure to flush the toilet twice. The maximum urine excretion occurs within 48 hours of the injection. In patients who are incontinent, plastic mattress covers and urine-absorbing undergarments are recommended; condom drainage or bladder catheterization also should be considered for anywhere from several days to a week after the injection. You do not need to alter your diet before or after the therapy.

Newer radionuclide agents are under investigation for the treatment of symptomatic bone metastases in men with mCRPC that appear to delay skeletal-related adverse events and increase overall survival in preliminary studies, coupled with a lower risk of a drop in white blood cell and platelet counts.

18. I hear the newer therapies are expensive. Will my insurance cover them?

Many of the pharmaceutical companies offer assistance programs to decrease the out-of-pocket expenses related to the medications for those who qualify.

Yes, the newer therapies are expensive, with costs ranging from $5,000 to $7,500 per month for the oral therapies, $3,342 to $7,200 per cycle for chemotherapy, and $31,000 per cycle for immunotherapy. However, most insurance companies and Medicare cover the majority of the cost of the medications. Many of the pharmaceutical companies offer assistance programs to decrease the out-of-pocket expenses related to the medications for those who qualify. For individuals without insurance, assistance programs are also available. If the out-of-pocket costs of the medication are concerning to you, talk to your doctor or contact the drug's assistance program to see what forms of assistance, if any, you qualify for.

19. I am depressed. Is that common? Is there any way to help cope with my worries?

The diagnosis of prostate cancer comes as a shock to most men. For those diagnosed with organ-confined cancer, there is the hope that the cancer can be cured by surgical or radiation-based therapies. However, for those who recur and/or those with extensive cancer not responsive to curative therapies, the hope for cure is not a reality. Instead, focus is placed on preventing the cancer from progressing. In individuals with CRPC, a rising PSA level and/or development of metastases can lead to fear, anger, confusion, and depression. It is not unusual to initially "retreat" from life as you absorb the reality of the situation and begin to gather more information and start to decide what therapy to try next. It is difficult to be optimistic about future treatments when other treatments have proven ineffective, and you may feel overwhelmed. If you find that you feel like a failure, are continuing to withdraw socially, feel that you are being punished, are thinking about committing suicide, feel helpless and can't make decisions, have lost interest in activities that once brought you pleasure, or are crying a lot, then you could be suffering from a more severe depression. This should be discussed with your doctor. Sometimes, when faced with such potentially overwhelming situations, you might need some assistance to help you regain control of your life and make decisions regarding your further treatment.

If you feel lost and overwhelmed by the therapies available, their risks and benefits, and the impact of these therapies on your quality of life, talk to your doctor. Information and education will help you understand the available options and decide which one is best for you. Some people find help in support groups. There are prostate cancer support groups. These often can be found at your local hospital and typically meet on a regular basis. Often, there are guest speakers at the support groups to address key concerns of the group, such as impact of therapy on quality of life, newer forms of therapy, and other issues. Prostate cancer support groups provide an informal setting to express one's concerns, ask questions, and share information with others. Frequently, spouses and significant others attend and are invited to discuss their concerns. Discussing some of your concerns with others who are going through or have gone through what you are experiencing could help alleviate some of your anxieties and help you focus on what questions you need to have answered by your doctor(s) as you make treatment decisions. To find out about your local prostate cancer support group, ask your **urologist**, oncologist, or local hospital. The American Cancer Society might also be able to help you identify a local prostate cancer support group.

The most important thing to do if you feel depressed and/or overwhelmed is to reach out and ask for help.

Urologist

A doctor that specializes in the evaluation and treatment of disease of the genitourinary tract in men and women.

20. My doctor mentioned clinical trials. What is a clinical trial? How do I find out what clinical trials are ongoing near where I live?

A clinical trial is a carefully planned **experiment** that is designed to evaluate the use of a treatment or a medication for an unproven use. Through the use of clinical trials, investigators assess newer ideas in the treatment of various diseases. There are three phases of clinical trials, each with a particular goal. Typically, when a new medication or therapy is being introduced, its evaluation proceeds in an orderly process through each of these trials.

Phase I trials are preliminary, short-duration studies that involve only a few patients. These studies are used to see whether the medication or therapy has any effect or any serious side effects. Phase II trials involve a larger number of patients and are designed to determine the most effective dose of the therapy and its side effects. Phase III trials involve large numbers of patients and compare the new therapy with the current standard or best available therapy.

To find out about clinical trials in your area, you can first start by asking your urologist and/or oncologist. You can also contact your local hospital and the nearest cancer center. The Prostate Cancer Foundation has a list of ongoing clinical trials in the United States on their website *www.pcf.org*.

Experiment

An untested or unproven treatment or approach to treatment.

Typically, when a new medication or therapy is being introduced, its evaluation proceeds in an orderly process through each of these trials.

47

A

Adrenal glands: Glands located above each kidney. These glands produce several different hormones, including sex hormones.

Alopecia: Partial or complete loss of hair from parts of the body where it normally grows (baldness).

American Urological Association (AUA): A professional association in the United States for urologists.

Androgen deprivation therapy (ADT): Therapy designed to lower the testosterone level in the body by preventing its production (most commonly, LHRH agonists/antagonists).

Androgen receptor: A structure within the cell where androgen (testosterone and DHT) binds and is translocated (moved) into the cell to stimulate cell growth through the production of various proteins.

Androgens: Hormones that are necessary for the development and function of the male sexual organs and male sexual characteristics (hair, voice change). Testosterone and DHT are two types.

Anemia: Decrease in the number of red blood cells.

Anti-androgen: A medication that eliminates or reduces the presence or activity of androgens.

Antibody: A molecule produced by the body that reacts with a specific antigen that induced its synthesis.

Antigen: A substance that stimulates the body to produce an antibody.

Antigen-presenting cell (APC): A cell (dendritic cell) that activates the immune system by processing and presenting antigen to specialized immune cells (T cells) to activate them to reject and destroy cancer cells.

Arthralgia: Joint pain.

Asthenia: Abnormal physical weakness or lack of energy.

B

Bilateral orchiectomy: Surgical removal of both testicles.

Bisphosphonate: A type of medication that is used to treat osteoporosis and the bone pain caused by some types of cancer.

Bone scan: A specialized nuclear medicine scan that allows doctors to detect changes in the bone that might be related to metastatic prostate cancer.

Brachytherapy: A form of radiation therapy in which radioactive pellets are inserted inside of the prostate.

C

Cancer: Abnormal and uncontrolled growth of cells in the body that can spread, injure areas of the body, and cause death.

Castration: The removal of both testicles (bilateral orchiectomy).

Castration resistant: Prostate cancer that progresses despite androgen deprivation therapy and resultant low (< 20–50 ng/dL) testosterone level.

Cell: The smallest unit of the body. Tissues in the body are made up of cells.

Chemotherapy: A treatment for cancer that uses powerful chemicals to weaken and destroy the cancer cells.

Chronic obstructive pulmonary disease (COPD): A group of lung diseases that block airflow and make breathing difficult.

Clinical trial: A carefully planned and regulated experiment to evaluate a treatment or medication (often a new drug) for an unproven use.

Computerized tomography/ computerized axial tomography (CT/ CAT) scan: A specialized X-ray study that allows doctors to visualize internal structures in cross-section to look for abnormalities.

CYP17 inhibitor: An inhibitor of an enzyme found in steroid-hormone-producing tissues, adrenal glands, testicles, and prostate cancer cells.

Cytokine: Any of a number of substances secreted by certain cells of the immune system that regulate responses to infection, immune responses, inflammation, and trauma.

D

Dendritic cells: See antigen-presenting cells.

Diagnosis: The identification of the cause or presence of a medical problem or disease.

Dihydrotestosterone (DHT): A breakdown product of testosterone that is more potent than testosterone.

Disease: Any change from or interruption of the normal structure or function of any part, organ, or system of the body that presents with characteristic symptoms and signs and whose cause and prognosis could be known or unknown.

Dual energy X-ray absorptiometry (DEXA) scan: An imaging system to assess bone mineral density.

E

Edema: Swelling caused by excess fluid trapped in the body's tissue.

Enzyme: A chemical that is produced by living cells that causes chemical reactions to occur without undergoing any changes itself.

Experiment: An untested or unproven treatment or approach to treatment.

F

Femur: The thigh bone.

Follicle stimulating hormone: A type of hormone produced by the pituitary that is involved in stimulating the production of sperm by the testicles.

Food and Drug Administration (FDA): The federal agency responsible for the approval of prescription medications in the United States.

Fusion protein: A protein created by joining two or more genes responsible for the production of separate individual proteins, resulting in a protein that has functional properties derived from each of the original proteins.

G

Gland: A structure or organ that produces substances that affect other areas of the body.

Granulocyte-macrophage colony-stimulating factor (GM-CSF): A protein secreted by several cells that stimulates the growth and development of various cells.

H

Hormones: Substances (estrogens and androgens) responsible for secondary sex characteristics (hair growth and voice change in men) and function of sexual organs.

Hormone therapy: The manipulation of a disease's natural history and symptoms through the use of hormones.

Hypocalcemia: Low calcium in the bloodstream.

Hypogonadism: In males, a condition in which the testicles do not produce enough testosterone.

Hypokalemia: Lower-than-normal potassium levels due to excessive excretion or inadequate uptake at the cellular level.

Hypothalamus: The region of brain that produces LHRH.

I

Immune system: A complex group of organs, tissues, blood cells, and substances that work to fight off infections, cancers, or foreign substances.

Immunotherapy: Treatment of disease by inducing, enhancing, or suppressing an immune response.

Indications: The reasons for undertaking a specific treatment, such as choice of therapy, surgical, medical, or other.

Intravenous: A term referring to liquid (medicine, fluids, etc.) that is administered through the veins.

L

LHRH agonist: A class of drugs that works at the level of the brain, which initially overstimulates the brain before suppressing the production of testosterone by the testicles. This short period of overstimulation can increase the testosterone level and cause bone pain in patients with bone metastases, known as the "flare phenomenon."

LHRH antagonist: A form of hormone therapy that works at the level of the brain to directly suppress the production of testosterone without initially raising the testosterone level. There is no flare reaction.

Lifestyle: The way a person chooses to live.

Lower respiratory tract infection: Acute infection involving bronchi (bronchitis) and/or lungs (pneumonia).

Lymph: A clear fluid that is found throughout the body. Lymph fluid helps fight infections.

Lymph node(s): Small, bean-shaped glands that are found throughout the body. Lymph fluid passes through the lymph nodes, which filter out bacteria, cancer cells, and toxic chemicals.

M

Magnetic resonance imaging (MRI): A study that is similar to a CT scan in that it allows one to see internal structures in detail, but different in that it does not involve radiation.

Maximum androgen blockade: The combination of androgen deprivation therapy and an androgen receptor blocker.

Metastases: See metastatic cancer.

Metastatic cancer: Cancer that has spread to another area in the body from the organ or structure in which it first arose.

Metastatic castration-resistant prostate cancer (mCRPC): Prostate cancer that continues to progress despite ADT and its resultant low (< 20–50 ng/dL) testosterone level and has spread to an area outside of the prostate gland, such as the bones or lymph nodes.

N

Noninvasive: Not requiring any incision or the insertion of an instrument or substance into the body.

O

Oncologist: A medical specialist who is trained to evaluate and treat cancer.

Orchiectomy: The surgical procedure that removes the testicle(s).

Organ: Tissues in the body (e.g., kidneys, bladder, heart) that work together to perform a specific function.

Osteoblast: A specialized cell that makes new bone.

Osteoclast: A specialized cell that breaks down bone.

Osteonecrosis of the jaw (ONJ): A severe bone disease that affects the bones of the jaw, the maxilla, and the mandible. It may occur in association with bisphosphonate and RANK-ligand inhibitor therapy.

Osteoporosis: Reduction in the amount of bone mass, leading to fractures after minimal trauma.

P

Paresthesia: Abnormal sensation, typically tingling or pricking, that could be due to nerve damage.

Performance status: In medicine (oncology and other fields), performance status is an attempt to quantify cancer patients' general well-being and activities of daily life. There are two commonly used scoring systems: the Karnofsky and the ECOG/WHO/Zubrod.

Pituitary gland: The region of the brain that produces LH.

Platelet: A cell found in large numbers in blood and involved in clotting.

Positron emission tomography (PET): A nuclear imaging technique that produces a three-dimensional image or picture of a functional process in the body.

Prednisone: A synthetic drug similar to corticosterone.

Pre-osteoclast: A specialized cell that develops into an osteoclast when stimulated by RANK-ligand.

Progression-free survival: The length of time during and after medication or treatment during which the disease being treated (cancer) does not get worse.

Prostatectomy: The removal of the prostate gland and the tissue surrounding it.

Prostatic acid phosphatase: An antigen produced by the prostate.

PSA nadir: The lowest value that the PSA level reaches during a particular treatment.

PSA progression: Rising PSA levels despite therapy to treat prostate cancer.

Q

Quality of life: An evaluation of healthy status relative to the patient's age, expectations, and physical and mental capabilities.

R

Radiation therapy: Use of radioactive beams or implants to kill cancer cells.

RANK-ligand (RANKL): A cytokine involved in the development of osteoclasts from pre-osteoclasts.

Receptor: A protein molecule located in either the outer edge of the cell or the inside of the cell. When substances bind to it, they direct the cell to do something.

Refractory: Resistant to therapy.

Risk: The chance or probability that an adverse outcome will occur.

S

Sensitivity: The probability that a diagnostic test can correctly identify the presence of a particular disease.

Sensory neuropathy: Damage to the nerves of the peripheral nervous system that can cause abnormal sensations, like tingling or a prick-like feeling.

Side effect: A reaction to a medication or treatment.

Sign: Objective evidence of a disease; something that the doctor identifies.

Single photon emission computerized tomography (SPECT): A type of nuclear imaging test that uses a radioactive substance and a special camera to create three-dimensional pictures.

Specificity: The probability that a diagnostic test can correctly identify the absence of disease.

Spinal cord compression: Compression of the spinal cord by bone, tumor, or other causes with symptoms ranging from temporary numbness to permanent paralysis of the body below the level of the compression.

Stomatitis: Inflammation of the lining of the mouth.

Symptom: Subjective evidence of a disease; something a patient describes, such as pain in the bones.

T

Taxane(s): A chemotherapy drug derived from the Yew plant that prevents cell growth by inhibiting special cell structures, called microtubules, which are involved in cell division.

Testicles: One of the two male reproductive organs that are located within the scrotum and produce testosterone and sperm.

Testosterone: The male hormone or androgen that is produced primarily by the testes and is needed for sexual function and fertility.

Thrombocytopenia: A decrease in the platelet count of the blood.

Total (maximal) androgen blockade: The total blockage of production and action of testosterone through surgery and/or medications.

U

Upper respiratory tract infection: An acute infection involving the nose, sinuses, and throat.

Ureters: The tubes that drain the urine from the kidneys to the bladder.

Urologist: A doctor that specializes in the evaluation and treatment of disease of the genitourinary tract in men and women.

X

X-ray: A type of high-energy radiation that can be used at low levels to make images of the internal structures of the body and at high levels for radiation therapy.

GLOSSARY

55

Note: Page numbers followed by "*f*" and "*t*" indicate figures and tables, respectively.

INDEX